A Complete Look at Hy

Underactive Thyroid Symptoms and Treatments

By: James M. Lowrance © 2008

INTRODUCTION:

Hypothyroidism is the medical term for an under-active thyroid gland. Hypothyroid disorders account for about 80% of thyroid disease cases, with the other 20% being hyperthyroid disorders (overactive thyroid). In this book, I will be addressing the subjects of symptoms, diagnosis and treatments for hypothyroidism. Within the chapters that follow, I will also be discussing blood tests and other diagnostic methods for detecting under-functioning thyroid glands and aspects of thyroid hormone replacement therapy. It is my hope that this e-book provides the reader with a general education on the subject of hypothyroidism.

TABLE OF CONTENTS:

CHAPTER ONE: Symptoms and Diagnosis of Hypothyroidism

CHAPTER TWO: Common Causes of Hypothyroidism

CHAPTER THREE: Treatment for Hypothyroidism

CHAPTER FOUR: The Pros and Cons of Hypothyroid Treatment

CHAPTER FIVE: My Personal Experience with Hypothyroidism

CHAPTER ONE

Symptoms and Diagnosis of Hypothyroidism

Thyroid diseases affect an estimated 28,000,000 Americans and 80% of these have "hypothyroidism" or a low-functioning thyroid gland. According to medical experts, including the AACE (American Association of Clinical Endocrinologists) about half of those with thyroid hormone imbalances, remain undiagnosed. This is likely due to a combination of both lack of diagnostic testing being ordered by doctors and a lack of public education in regard to recognizing hypothyroid and hyperthyroid symptoms. Two major thyroid hormones, called T-3 (triiodothyronine) and T-4 (thyroxine), regulate the metabolism of every cell of our body. When the thyroid gland produces a lack of these, due to hindrance from a disease process it is experiencing or for any other reason, the body experiences "hypothyroidism", resulting in a slowed-down metabolism (reduced energy within all bodily cells).

Americans should become better educated in regard to the symptoms of hypothyroidism and the tests ordered for diagnosing it, so that they can recognize it and receive the needed treatment from a licensed physician. One way in which public awareness is being gained, is via "Thyroid Awareness Month", which occurs each year, during the month of January. Medical groups and patient advocates use the month to place extra push behind spreading information to the general population in regard to recognizing thyroid disorders, which are more common than diabetes and heart disease combined.

Symptoms of Hypothyroidism

When a person is experiencing bodily-symptoms they may suspect hypothyroidism if one or more of them match the following, which are commonly listed for an under-active thyroid gland:

- Feeling cold in warm temperatures

- Dry skin and brittle fingernails

- Hair that becomes brittle and breaks off or falls out

- Thinning of the eyebrows and loss of the outer 1/3 portion of them

- Unexplained weight gain with no diet change

- Constipation

- Slowed heart rate and breathing

- Depression

- Physical tiredness/fatigue

- Feeling a fullness or tightness in the throat (a sign of goiter)

If you experience any of these symptoms, you should see your doctor and describe them to him/her, in-detail and ask if blood tests might be needed to diagnose or rule out the problem as being hypothyroidism, in addition to other tests that might be recommended.

Other medical conditions can mimic hypothyroidism, including diabetes, nutritional deficiencies and sex hormone imbalances and so a qualified doctor can determine the testing that is needed. Even with this being the fact, patient-input regarding testing that may be needed, should be welcomed by doctors who want to see a reasonable degree of proactiveness from their patients and who see them as partners in their ongoing health care.

Tests for Hypothyroidism

While the symptoms and signs listed previously, point to possible thyroid disease and specifically to potential hypothyroidism, it is important once they are recognized as signs of a slowed metabolism, to have all of the proper blood tests ordered. Blood testing is the single most effective method, for detecting many common health disorders and diseases that exists in the field of professional medicine and this is certainly true of detecting thyroid dysfunction as well.

Thorough-evaluation thyroid testing comes in a grouping of tests called a "thyroid panel".

These tests of thyroid hormone levels, include a test of the "TSH" level, which is a pituitary hormone ("Thyroid Stimulating Hormone" -- also called "thyrotropin") that the master endocrine brain-gland sends to the thyroid gland, stimulating it to produce the correct amount of thyroid hormones that are needed by the body to regulate metabolism. This is the reason it is called a "stimulating hormone" and when it becomes elevated above the normal range, this means the thyroid is falling behind in producing adequate hormones to supply the body. Some doctors actually use the TSH alone, in testing patients for hypothyroidism and also for an overactive thyroid (hyperthyroidism) because of its sensitivity in detecting abnormal thyroid function earlier than any other thyroid function test. This pituitary hormone will sometimes detect hypothyroidism, even before the actual thyroid hormones do (before the T-3 and T-4 fall outside of normal limits).

Differences between Diagnostic and Treatment TSH

I have received a number of e-mails from thyroid patients responding to articles I have written over the years, which were on the subject of "TSH blood testing". They are complaining of not feeling well, in spite of being on thyroid medication and have included their most recent, follow-up lab results in their e-mails to me. In almost every one of these, their TSH levels are within the "normal" range for diagnosing hypothyroidism but they are not within the normal range for treating hypothyroidism and incredibly, they are stating that their Doctors are telling them that there is no difference between the two. There is a difference between the two however; and we only need to look at reliable medical sources to recognize this fact.

The "diagnostic" TSH levels, as revised and recommended by the AACE, in 2002 are roughly 0.3 to 3.0.

The "treatment" TSH level they recommend, is 1.0 to 2.0 for titrating hormone replacement therapy (adjusting thyroid medication levels in hypothyroid patients) however, many patients feel better, at the 1.0 and even down to the lowest TSH normal level of just above 0.3. Some patients even need a TSH that is slightly below the normal treatment level, due to slightly sluggish pituitary function that causes a TSH level that doesn't accurately represent the actual thyroid hormone levels but these cases require close monitoring by their Doctors. When the pituitary gland is actually under functioning, this is referred to as "hypopituitarism" however, some people may have subclinical forms of this problem that in some cases eventually causes a condition called "Central Hypothyroidism" (more on this subject in a succeeding chapter). For the general population of hypothyroid patients, the treatment range of 1.0 to 2.0 is the standard, among the top thyroid doctors .

Unfortunately, if a Doctor uses the diagnostic TSH range, a patient may be receiving inadequate treatment because this would mean that he or she would recognize even the highest-normal TSH, as being sufficient treatment, when it is most often not adequate for restoring a normal metabolism. For example, if a patient is treated on thyroid hormone replacement medication and their treatment dose only suppresses their TSH down to 3.0, the Doctor who is not using the treatment TSH guideline but rather the diagnostic range, will recognize this level as being sufficient and the patient may continue to experience hypothyroid symptoms. This scenario is worsened, when the blood testing lab a Doctor is using, still abides by the old "diagnostic" TSH level of 0.5 to 5.0, revised by the AACE, in 2002 as previously mentioned, that helps diagnose developing hypothyroidism, being the current 0.3 to 3.0. Many labs have adjusted their ranges but some have set their high-normal cut-off value, somewhere between the old range and the revised one, such as having an upper-limit of "4.0". This is still considerable improvement over the former 5.0 and 6.0 values that most labs formerly adhered-to.

During my first two years of treatment for hypothyroidism, my first Doctor kept my TSH between 3.01 and 4.95 and stated that even that higher level was a "perfect reading". In reality, it was not only inadequate thyroid dosing, but I was virtually spinning-my-wheels and getting very little accomplished in reducing my hypothyroid symptoms. Once finding a better-informed Doctor, who placed me on combination T-4/T-3 replacement hormone medication and dosing me, to reduce my TSH level to between 0.5 and 1.0, I felt better than I had in my first three years of treatment.

The Endocrinologist, who treats me currently, agrees with other thyroid specialists who treat patients optimally, by getting their TSH levels down to lowest normal values. A thyroid patient forum I previously posted at a great deal, that has a Board Certified Endocrinologist answering questions on, repeatedly confirmed that his patients felt better with a TSH around 1.0 and that many of them he replaced with doses that would suppress their TSH levels down to between 0.5 and 1.0.

Thyroid Panels

A "thyroid panel" will also include a test of the actual thyroid hormone levels, which are the "T-4," also called the "thyroxine level", containing four iodine molecules and the "T-3," also called the "triiodothyronine level", containing three iodine molecules. The T-4 is referred to in medical sources as a "reserve hormone" and as a "precursor hormone" and while it helps the body with metabolism at the tissue-level, it also converts into the more active T-3 hormone, which is several times more powerful than the T-4 hormone (by 5 to 10 times) and is more active in regulating the body's metabolism. Either one of these two hormones or a combination of the two being found low in the blood, indicates hypothyroidism. If the TSH is also high, with either of these being low, this, too, indicates hypothyroidism. Even if these two thyroid hormones are in the normal range but TSH is elevated, this too can indicate hypothyroidism.

The T-4 and T-3 blood tests come in a variety of different versions, such as the "totals" of each, the "free" levels of each or may be combined in tests called the "FTI Index" or the "T-7".

There is also one called the "T-3 Uptake". All of these help to determine thyroid hormone production levels and all of them have lab ranges with a "below-normal" indicating hypothyroidism and an "above-normal" indicating hyperthyroidism.

A 24 hour Thyroid Uptake Scan is another test of thyroid function that doctors sometimes use to detect hypothyroidism (more frequent used for diagnosing hyperthyroid disorders). The patient being tested will receive a dose of radioactive iodine, administered by a doctor or a lab technician, that is absorbed by the thyroid gland. The radiological imaging that follows reveals how well the thyroid is functioning, by highlighting the tissues within the gland. It does this by revealing how well iodine is absorbed by the gland and whether this is occurring evenly or if part of the gland is failing. An Uptake Scan can determine how well the thyroid functions to a highly accurate estimated percentage-level.

CHAPTER TWO

Common Causes of Hypothyroidism

When it is determined that a patient has hypothyroidism, the doctor will then further investigate to find the cause of the low functioning thyroid gland. The most common cause found in patients with hypothyroidism in the industrialized countries of the world, is an immune system response that is referred to as "thyroid autoimmunity". "Hashimoto's thyroiditis" is the usual term applied to this cause although, there are other variations, such as "Ord's thyroiditis" (the latter being a more common finding in countries of the UK). The condition is also medically known as "chronic lymphocytic thyroiditis" and results in a slow destruction of the gland, rendering it unable to provide the body with ample amounts of thyroid hormones. Some Hashimoto's patients also experience goiters but they are usually mild, while those with Ord's actually see their thyroid glands shrink (atrophy) over time.

Hashimoto's Thyroiditis

The majority of patients with both hypothyroidism (under-active thyroid) and hyperthyroidism (overactive thyroid) are experiencing autoimmune diseases that cause these conditions. When the autoimmune disease of the thyroid causes hyperthyroidism, it is called "Grave's Disease". I discuss the symptoms, causes, diagnosis and treatments for hyperthyroid conditions, in the book titled ***"A Complete Look at Hyperthyroidism"***.

The immune system normally sends out antibodies, which are killer cells designed to eradicate foreign invaders from the body that can make us sick. These invaders include viruses, bacteria and allergens. The purpose of antibodies is to seek these out and to destroy them, to prevent our bodies from becoming ill. The problem with "thyroid antibodies" is that, like other antibodies that cause autoimmune diseases, they are eventually directed against normal tissues such as the thyroid gland as if it is one of these invaders. It is a case of mistaken identity that over time causes damage to the thyroid gland via ongoing cell death.

Eventually, the antibodies will actually kill-out the thyroid gland completely over time, turning its healthy tissue into an unhealthy type that no longer absorbs iodine from the diet, in order to manufacture its metabolism-regulating hormones.

As previously-mentioned, thyroid autoimmunity means your gland is being attacked by antibodies that are sent from the immune system that have the goal of destroying it. This autoimmune process not only damages the thyroid gland but it also causes inflammation within it, which is where the "thyroiditis" term comes from. The antibodies can also serve to block some of the thyroid hormone produced by the gland, so that it doesn't do the job it needs to, even when there is near-ample levels available in the body. Patients can have varying symptoms at the early stage of autoimmune hypothyroidism, such as the subclinical types (not full blown) and the overt types (full blown).

As mentioned earlier, it is the most common cause of a low functioning thyroid in many industrialized countries of the world, including the US, second only to iodine deficiency hypothyroidism which is more prominent in less-developed countries that all-combined, represent a majority of the world-population.

Diagnosis of Hashimoto's Thyroiditis

Patients suspected of having this autoimmune form of thyroid disease, need to be tested for thyroid antibodies, in addition to being tested for low levels of thyroid hormone. In some cases, these antibody tests can reveal that autoimmune thyroid disease is going on, in patients with normal range thyroid hormone levels. The tests that help detect Hashimoto's thyroiditis, are the "anti-TPO" (anti-thyroidperoxidase) and the "anti-TG" (anti-thyroglobulin) and sometimes also the "TSI" antibodies (thyroid stimulating immunoglogulin), although these latter mentioned ones are more commonly found positive in patients with Graves' disease.

People with developing autoimmune hypothyroidism (Hashimoto's thyroiditis), can have elevated antibody levels that cause them a degree of symptoms, even when thyroid hormones levels fall within normal-range.

Medical research articles by reputable medical groups, state this fact regarding the disease process itself, involving thyroid antibodies as being a factor in causing symptoms in Hashimoto's patients. These research articles conclude that elevated levels of these immune cells can cause fibromyalgia and other rheumatic types of symptoms in persons with only sub-clinical hypothyroidism. Some of these articles also state that autoimmune thyroid disease can have a degree of systemic (system-wide) effect, so that the immune system response affects not only the thyroid gland area but other parts of the body as well.

Following is a quote from an article published on the PubMed website (U.S. National Institutes of Health), stating that the autoimmunity aspect of the disease, rather than abnormal thyroid hormone levels alone, are what contribute to the symptoms of Hasihimoto's disease:

"A variety of rheumatic manifestations have been described in association with autoimmune thyroiditis. In the past, most of these manifestations were attributed to the underlying thyroid dysfunction, in particular hypothyroidism. However, a responsibility of the mechanisms involved in the autoimmunity rather than a direct action of thyroid hormones seems supported by the evidences that some rheumatic manifestations may occur even in euthyroid patients, or that they are more frequent in hypothyroid patient with autoimmune thyroiditis than in those without this disease.

Rheumatic manifestations could be sometimes attributable to the autoimmune rheumatic diseases frequently associated with autoimmune thyroiditis, such as Sjögren's syndrome, rheumatoid arthritis, systemic lupus erythematosus, or scleroderma. Among the most important or frequent rheumatic manifestations there are a mild non-erosive variety of arthritis, polyarthralgia, myalgia, and sicca syndrome without a true Sjögren's syndrome.

Although the possible pathogenesis of these manifestations is not completely established, some hypotheses may be proposed, including a role of autoantibodies characteristics of autoimmune thyroiditis, a possible overlap between autoimmune thyroiditis and some autoimmune rheumatic diseases, and a systemic inflammatory reaction associated with thyroiditis."

(From the research article titled: "Chronic autoimmune thyroiditis and rheumatic manifestations." - Online Link Location: http://www.ncbi.nlm.nih.gov/pubmed/15288851)

Hashitoxicosis

Patients with Hashimoto's thyroiditis can also go through phases of temporary hyperthyroidism, before the onset of progressive hypothyroidism sets in and the term for this related condition is "Hashitoxicosis".

These patients are the ones mentioned previously, who might need to be blood tested for TSI antibodies because the hyperthyroid phases they go through are due to having some elevation of these antibodies, that normally cause Grave's Disease (autoimmune hyperthyroidism), in addition to the ones that cause Hashimoto's thyroiditis (Anti-TPO and Anti-TG).

Here is a quote from an online resource in regard to Hashitoxicosis:

"Hashitoxicosis is an autoimmune thyroid disorder, in which individuals with autoimmune hypothyrodism, usually Hashimoto's thyroiditis (HT), experience intermittent or sporadic periods where they also have symptoms of hyperthyrodism." (Grave's Disease and Hyperthyroidism Wiki)

You could almost say that these patients are suffering from Grave's and Hashimoto's, simultaneously.

Even without having the TSI antibodies present, Hashimoto's patients can experience flares of thyroiditis (spells of increased thyroid inflammation), which can also cause mild hyperthyroid type symptoms that are not as severe as those caused by Hashitoxicosis but that are still concerning. Not all medical sources agree on this aspect and some believe that Hashitoxicosis can only be identified as such if hyperthyroid symptoms are severe, rather than mild, as can be the case with episodes of thyroiditis.

Central Hypothyroidism

Hypothyroidism can also be caused by a failure in the chain of communication between the glands that work in-sync with each other and that normally results in the proper release of thyroid hormone from the thyroid gland. The "pituitary gland", a major brain-gland actually sends messages to the thyroid gland using the messenger hormone called "TSH".

If there is a problem within the pituitary gland in being able to stimulate the thyroid, such as an obstructive tumor that develops within it, causing it to also be low functioning (hypopituitarism), the cause would then be referred to as "Central Hypothyroidism".

Other Secondary Causes

In more complicated cases, hypothyroidism might be secondary to another disease process in the body, in which case, extensive blood testing of all types may need to be undertaken to determine the underlying cause of the thyroid hormone imbalance or what is also referred to as "Secondary Hypothyroidism".

Certain types of illnesses and severe, chronic stress, can cause the body to convert too much of the T-4 hormone into an inactive form of hormone called "Reverse T-3" (T-4 normally converts into adequate amounts of the active T-3), which will cause a person to experience a type of "hypothyroidism", due to low T-3 hormone in the body.

This type of hypothyroidism that is secondary to an illness or from severe stress in the body is also referred to as "Sick Euthyroid Syndrome" or "low T-3 Syndrome" and is also sometimes referred to as "Wilson's Temperature Syndrome". It is usually a temporary form of hypothyroidism that can be corrected with short term T-3 hormone replacement therapy. This type of hypothyroidism is rare compared to the types that are caused by a diseased thyroid gland or "primary hypothyroidism".

Postpartum Hypothyroidism

When women experience low thyroid hormone after pregnancy, following giving birth, the term for this type of under-active thyroid is "postpartum hypothyroidism". This type happens in about 10% of new mothers within 12 months of giving birth and for some it improves on its own, without treatment. Others may require short-term treatment with thyroid hormone replacement.

If the hypothyroidism that is triggered by pregnancy is the autoimmune type, the treatment for it will likely be life-long and the pregnancy simply brought the disease to the surface, which would have eventually manifested on its own over time.

Iodine Deficiency Hypothyroidism

One common acquired type of hypothyroidism that occurs in countries where diets are low in iodine is referred to as "iodine deficiency hypothyroidism". This type is rare in industrialized countries, so is more common in those considered to be "third world countries" (less developed and less industrialized and usually poverty level).

You don't often hear of people getting their iodine levels checked because iodine doesn't necessarily tell you anything about your thyroid function. The iodine level in the body can fluctuate considerably, due to what is in your diet (i.e. consuming high iodine foods like kelp etc...) or because of supplements you take that contain iodine.

The real tests of thyroid function are the actual thyroid hormone levels; T-4 and T-3 (preferably the "free levels") and the TSH level which is the pituitary hormone previously discussed, that is highly sensitive in monitoring thyroid function via blood testing.

In regard to high iodine content foods or supplements containing iodine, I suggest not consuming these for several days before being evaluated for thyroid function via blood testing because iodine can work adversely in some people with autoimmune thyroid disease. It can cause fluctuations in thyroid antibodies and hormone levels, giving a false impression of how a patients thyroid function is actually running. Iodine is the treatment for hypothyroidism caused by iodine deficiency but this type is almost non-existent in industrialized countries that manufacture iodized table salt. While there is some disagreement regarding this fact, it is believed that use of iodized salt alone usually contains as much iodine as average, healthy people need for proper thyroid function.

Following Thyroid Removal

Hyperthyroid patients, who have their thyroid glands either surgically removed (thyroidectomy) or destroyed by a process called "Radioactive Iodine Ablation", to halt their hyperthyroidism, will afterward become hypothyroid, with their glands no longer being present to manufacture thyroid hormones. They will afterward have to be given thyroid hormone replacement therapy just as patients who become hypothyroid due to any of the other previously listed reasons.

CHAPTER THREE

Treatment for Hypothyroidism

The treatment for hypothyroidism is simply to "replace" the low hormone levels and to restore what is needed by the body to regain a normal metabolism (rate at which the body uses energy from food, water and oxygen). This is done by giving the patient "thyroid hormone replacement medication". The Doctor will prescribe a starting dose for the patient and do follow-up blood re-testing to adjust the dose to the correct level over time, which is called "titrating" the dose -- the goal being to reach the most optimized levels possible.

Most patients with hypothyroidism are prescribed a T-4 only brand of thyroid hormone medication (e.i. Synthroid and brands of Levothyroxine) and the also needed T-3 hormone is converted from it, within the body successfully. In patients with a less-common problem called "impaired conversion" however, a T-4 only hormone medication will not supply them with adequate T-3 that is also needed in the body.

If this problem exists, it will be evident by their blood test results that monitor their dose. If a patient's T-4 to T-3 ratio is off too much they may need a thyroid hormone replacement medication that contains both T-4 and T-3 hormones (e.i. Armour Thyroid or Thyrolar) or they may need the addition of a T-3 medication (e.i. Cytomel) to the T-4 only brand they are already taking. There are also people who by taking a T-4/T-3 combination drug, elevate their Free T-3 level too high and have to be switched to a T-4 only medication. This is why it is important for hypothyroid patients to be treated by qualified doctors, who can determine the type of thyroid hormone medication that is best-suited for them.

Armour Thyroid Vs Other Natural Hypothyroidism Treatments

"Armour Thyroid" brand of prescribed hypothyroid therapy medication has a set dose of hormone, just like synthetic does. It contains 38mcg of T-4 (levothyroxin) 9mcg of T-3 (liothyronine) per each grain (60mg tablet).

The only change the medication makes once it enters the body is that the T-4 in it, will partially convert into more T-3, if the body determines it needs more. The other change would be the percent of absorption of it that can be affected by other things a patient is consuming at the time of taking their dose. Taking calcium or iron for example, within 6-hours of taking thyroid medication (either type), can limit its absorption in the body, as can too much dietary fiber, so these need to be consumed about 6 hours apart from taking the daily thyroid hormone dose.

There has been ongoing misinformation being published, in regard to the Armour brand not being consistent in doses however, Forest Pharmaceuticals, the manufacturer, has been cleared by the FDA for not having dosage inconsistencies within their tablets. Synthroid recently had to go through the same scrutiny and approval regarding pill-dose accuracy and so these accusations regarding dose-inconsistencies that sometime arise are likely fueled by pharmaceutical wars for market shares, more than anything else.

The Forest Company, who makes Armour, also makes synthetic T-4, just like Knoll Pharmaceuticals, the maker of Synthroid does. They also make a combo synthetic T-4 & T-3 combo (Thyrolar).

I am not recommending Armour over Synthroid because I believe some patients do better on Synthroid, however, I also believe Armour is given an undeserved "bad rap", by Doctors who are simply parroting what the Pharmaceutical companies are telling them. The fact is that Synthroid has had bad press on it at times, just as Armour has. I maintain my own belief that patients need trial-regimens of the opposite type medication, if they are tried on one and are not having success with it, via adequate or optimal symptom relief.

Prescribed thyroid hormones take-over for the thyroid gland, so that it atrophies (stops working) and this is actually the whole point of thyroid hormone replacement therapy. If a person waits until the thyroid gland completely stops functioning before starting thyroid medication, they risk serious health issues or even death by myxedema coma.

This is the dilemma, even for Doctors, in knowing at what point to actually start mildly-hypothyroid patients on hormone replacement because it always results in the eventual shut down of their own thyroid glands.

Symptoms are one of the most important reasons medication needs to be started but also, to help reduce elevated thyroid antibody levels (this sometimes takes years to achieve optimally) and to prevent goiter (swelling) and nodules (tumor-like growths) from developing within the gland and so we can see that there are multiple reasons for starting medication in patients with developing hypothyroidism.

Many medical resources state that thyroid medications help to reduce antibodies over time (opposite of what others claim – that it can increase them). If antibody levels increase despite being on medication, this does not necessarily mean the medication is the cause of this but it could also be due to thyroiditis flares that happen commonly with autoimmune hypothyroid disease.

The point to all this being that it is unavoidable to take hormone replacement medication if you have Hashimoto's disease as the cause of hypothyroidism because it is very rarely ever reversed and it is usually progressive.

Thyroid Boosters versus Hormone Replacement

There are companies who market non-prescription natural "thyroid supplements" and they know many Doctors will not approve these in combination with thyroid hormone replacement and so they claim these should be taken <u>instead</u> of a medically prescribed drug. It's very possible that these help to boost thyroid function for a while but to claim they will reverse autoimmune thyroid disease is false. If there were supplements that could do this, medical research would have discovered it many years ago.

While I believe there are natural supplements that can definitely improve a person's thyroid function, I do not believe they can replace thyroid hormone replacement medications, needed by patients with advanced disease of the gland that has already caused moderate or overt hypothyroidism. It is my opinion, and one I know also agrees with that of most medical professionals, that trying to replace thyroid hormone medication, containing actual thyroid hormone with a supplement containing no thyroid hormone, or an inconsistent amount, could actually be dangerous. Lack of thyroid hormone in the body, must be replaced and a patient cannot depend upon a supplement instead, that is supposed to increase thyroid function when the thyroid has lost ground that cannot be regained, once it is permanently damaged due to a disease process.

One has to be careful to read the ingredients of supplements being considered because Endocrinologists often warn patients that these "thyroid supplements" that contain no hormone, will not treat hypothyroidism and some contain ingredients that may actually work adversely with thyroid medications, including iodine.

With the fact of autoimmune thyroid disease not being able to be reversed except in very rare cases, this would mean that even if those supplements worked to help strengthen the thyroid gland, how long would this improvement last? If the thyroid starts going downhill again once these supplements were stopped, this would mean they would have to be lifelong treatment as well. If antibodies continued to attack the thyroid while one is on these non-hormone supplements, the gland would still eventually become so damaged over time, that there is no way they could continue to restore its function.

Best TSH Treatment Level

As briefly mentioned previously, the AACE (Endocrine Society/Thyroid Specialists) and other medical authorities recommend that hypothyroid patient's TSH levels while on thyroid hormone replacement medication, be suppressed down to between "1.0 and 2.0". The TSH level rises, when thyroid hormone decreases and it falls when the thyroid hormone levels increase.

If a patient's TSH is not kept below 2.0, they risk continued hypothyroid symptoms (patients can vary in their needs) and if it is brought significantly below 1.0, they risk patients developing hyperthyroid symptoms (dose-induced thyrotoxicity). Some Endocrinologists actually keep some patient's TSH levels between, "0.3 to 1.0" (lowest normal) if they feel the patient has a slightly sluggish pituitary gland or is simply a patient who does not fit into the general population in regard to their TSH level. These type cases, take careful monitoring by treating doctors as also previously mentioned.

CHAPTER FOUR

The Pros and Cons of Hypothyroid Treatment

Patients, who are diagnosed with hypothyroidism and are being treated for it with hormone replacement therapy, can sometimes have other imbalances that hinder the effectiveness of their treatment. Things such as adrenal hormones being low or low levels of ferritin/iron, Vitamin B-12 etc... (elements needed for strong blood), can cause thyroid hormone treatment, to be less effective in patients with imbalances of these and this is why thorough blood testing of all major nutritional levels may need to be done, to find any problems that prevent the treatment from working as well.

Tips for Taking Thyroid Hormone Medication for Best Results

People taking thyroid hormone replacement medication for hypothyroidism need to follow a set-routine for taking their daily dose. Hormone therapy can have a delicate balance and even small variations in the levels within the body can greatly affect how well a patient feels.

The steps below help to insure the best results from thyroid hormone replacement therapy.

Take your thyroid hormone medication on an empty stomach, with plenty of water. Many patients find it easier to take their thyroid medication on an empty stomach by doing so first thing in the morning before having breakfast. Once the medication has been taken, it is recommended that a patient wait at least 30 minutes before eating, to allow the medication time to be absorbed adequately within the digestive tract. Taking the medication with a full glass of water also helps with digestion and absorption of the medication.

Take your thyroid hormone medication at the same time each day. When you take your thyroid medication at the same time each day, this helps your hormone levels remain more stable than if you take it at different times each day. Most thyroid medications have a long half-life of several days (those containing T3 have a half-life of only a few hours).

Even very small changes in the rhythm of your dosage can affect the way you feel. According to the manufacturers of thyroid medications, the hormone will peak in the body at a certain time after ingesting it and then remain stable for a period of time and afterward have a slightly lowered effect. A patient will want to see the peak and stable effects during the day and the lowered effect toward the end of the day, as time for rest and sleep arrives after daily of activities.

If you take vitamins or supplements containing iron or calcium, be sure to take them six hours apart from your thyroid medication dose. As previously-mentioned, these two supplements can have a negative effect on thyroid hormone medication, by preventing it from fully absorbing in the body, if they are taken at the same time or too-close to the time of the hormone replacement dose. To prevent malabsorption, it is recommended that you take these supplements at least six hours apart from your thyroid medication each day (some sources suggest eight hours as added precaution).

Some patients take their thyroid medication in the morning on an empty stomach and will take their supplements containing iron and/or calcium after lunch, six hours later, to prevent this problem.

When you have blood retests of your thyroid hormone levels, take your medication at the same time, to correlate with each blood draw. Some patients on the day of a blood draw (to retest their thyroid hormone levels) will skip their thyroid medication dose until after their blood is drawn. Other patients will take their thyroid medication dose before the blood draw but will make sure the blood is drawn at the same time for each retest, to make sure levels are consistent in correlation with it. It really is not that important which method one may use, as long as they do-so consistently for each blood draw to retest their thyroid hormone levels while being treated for hypothyroidism.

Never adjust your own thyroid medication dose. There can be times when hypothyroid symptoms may manifest themselves despite the fact that you are taking your thyroid medication properly.

This might make some patients believe that a slight increase in their dose that day would help to relieve these symptoms, and consequently they are tempted to take it upon themselves to increase their dose. This is never a good idea, without the consent and supervision of a doctor. Even small adjustments in a prescribed dose can alter hormone levels in the body, for days at a time. If a patient seems to be experiencing symptoms of low thyroid hormone or those of an overactive thyroid (too much hormone), they should report these to their doctor for instructions on adjusting their medication or in making an office visit for further evaluation of their treatment.

Hypothyroid Hormone Therapy Always Perfect?

I receive e-mails often from treated hypothyroid patients, in fact one I received from a woman recently who had not yet been started on treatment, stating that she repeatedly went to Doctors with the full array of hypothyroid symptoms and all of her thyroid hormone levels, including TSH were all within the normal range, even with repeated testing.

She finally demanded antibody tests and her Doctor said that the results of these "were off the map", meaning they were very highly elevated, so he went ahead and placed her on thyroid medication because of her symptoms.

Many medical information sources state that Hashimoto's thyroiditis does not cause symptoms, only the resulting hypothyroidism, once detectable by abnormal thyroid hormone blood tests will cause symptoms. In my experience in corresponding with many hypothyroid patients by email and as a thyroid disease forum moderator, I have found that far too many untreated patients report symptoms before hormone levels fall outside the normal range, for this to be an uncommon experience. This also means that the same disease that results in already-treated patient's hypothyroidism can potentially continue to cause a degree of symptoms when hormone levels are corrected back into the normal range, even at optimal levels.

The description of expected results from thyroid medications, from those who state that thyroid autoimmunity is not a factor in symptoms, describe it in almost miraculous or magical terms such as one I read recently that stated to the effect; "once on thyroid hormone medication, any symptoms a patient has will resolve and the patient will return to normal within a few weeks". Improvement, yes! Symptoms completely resolved and a return to normal, not in all cases! A large percent of patients may see near-perfect results but for many, there is ongoing struggle with a degree of symptoms because autoimmune thyroiditis is a disease and is not cured by correcting the hypothyroidism that results from it, in fact no cure has yet been discovered.

We are thankful and grateful for the results we do experience from hormone replacement therapy but many in the medical community, need to be realistic with patients who can feel let down by anything less than what they are told will happen. If perfect-relief is not experienced, the patient is told "it is not their thyroid" and usually they will then be diagnosed with psychosomatic or emotional problems.

Emotions may very well be some of the symptoms that do not resolve completely with hypothyroid treatment. It is only fair to the patient however, for the emotional diagnosis to be described as being "thyroid related" if the symptoms manifested with their thyroid disease and the patient had no prior problems with them before the disease-onset. This may also be opportunity for the doctor to give the patient a trial of a different prescribed hormone, to see if it has better success with relieving their unresolved emotional symptoms.

I have also read some articles recently stating to the effect that "patients who do not see their symptoms resolve once optimized on thyroid hormone medication, are simply experiencing added stress and worry from the reality of having the disease". These are the type things that have given me a passion for this particular aspect of misinformation. It's hard to sit-still while literally thousands of thyroid patients are pegged with these unfair descriptions that simply are not true in most cases.

You would think from some of these descriptions, that this disease is just a mild condition similar to a cold, that is easily treatable and that seldom ever causes ongoing problems once treated. This is why research articles about "the role of thyroid autoimmunity" in symptoms both physical and emotional and the "Health Related Quality of Life of Thyroid Patients" surveys that are being conducted are so important in my opinion.

Too many medical sources and thyroid medication manufacturers, still state simply that once a patient with Hashimoto's-hypothyroidism for example, is on replacement hormone, they will get better and no longer suffer symptoms, after about 6-weeks or so on a dose of the hormone medication. The fact is however, that many patients need several dose adjustments before reaching the proper level of replacement that restores them to a eutyhroid (normalized) state.

This can take a process of many months as determined by each individual case and treating doctors should inform patients of this possibility. Patients should also be informed of the fact that "thyroid autoimmunity" has potential to contribute to symptoms in some patients, apart from corrected thyroid hormone levels.

While most patients do see significant improvement, many still suffer a degree of symptoms, no matter how optimized their treatment is because the medication does not cure the underlying autoimmune disease that causes the thyroid imbalance. For this reason, patients should not be patronized and made to feel ridiculous or have it implied to them that they are hypochondriacs or experiencing psychosomatic symptoms, simply because they do not see complete relief of symptoms from thyroid replacement hormone therapy.

CHAPTER FIVE

My Personal Experience with Hypothyroidism

My story started at age 40, in early 2003, when I crashed into severe symptoms of thyroid disease and had no idea what it was. Mine followed a severe period of stress, which according to many patient-testimonials and medical research articles, can be a trigger for underlying thyroid disease to surface.

I visited a doctor who was filling-in for my regular doctor and she immediately diagnosed me with Generalized Anxiety Disorder and prescribed me an antidepressant, an anti-anxiety medication and a beta-blocker to control my adrenaline surges. My symptoms were: fatigue, post exertion malaise, brain fog, very dry skin, anxiety, depression, severe sweating, weight loss (rapid and temporary), joint aches and my hair was starting to break off and fall out in small amounts. The symptoms scared me out of my wits!

I knew beyond a doubt that there were more than emotions going on in my body, so I demanded a blood draw and asked for my thyroid hormones, glucose and blood counts to be tested. I had the blood drawn before I started the antidepressant that was prescribed. The Hospital lost my lab results for over a month and didn't bother to tell me and when I called about them after waiting to hear about my results through my Doctor's office, they said everything looked great and not to worry about it.

My own doctor, who was gone at the time I made the visit the fill-in doctor, returned for a short period of time before leaving again to become a missionary doctor in a foreign country. Just before he left, he was able to locate my lab results and wrote me a review letter in regard to them. His first sentence stated: "Your lab tests indicate you are low on thyroid hormone". He also pointed out that I was borderline diabetic. The hospital staff, who said my tests were normal, made me realize that you cannot take the word of someone other than a doctor in regard to medical issues and you need to see all of your own lab results (request copies – because you are entitled to them by law).

My TSH on the lab results, was elevated at "8.3" (lab range - 0.4 to 4.5) and my T-3 Uptake was several points below normal. I followed up with tests that revealed my hypothyroidism to be caused by Hashimoto's thyroiditis. My TG antibodies were at "537" (normal range <40) and my TPO antibodies were "120" (normal range <35). I also found through other lab testing that my cortisol levels were low (adrenal fatigue) but an ACTH Stimulation test ruled out true (full blown) adrenal insufficiency.

I was started on Synthroid (synthetic T4) in 2003 and later switched to Armour Thyroid (natural T4 and T3) in 2004. My doctor who switched me thought I might be one of the rare cases of "inadequate T-4 to T-3 conversion" (a condition I mention briefly in a previous chapter) but actually I was under-dosed on the Synthroid. Regardless, I do well on Armour and now take 2.5 grains (150mg). I also take vitamins and supplements that help the adrenal fatigue that flares when I'm physically overactive or experiencing high stressor levels and/or prolonged stress.

I was also diagnosed with Non-alcoholic Fatty Liver Disease, caused by Metabolic Syndrome (an insulin resistance type condition). I continue to work on weight loss/control and improved diet, to avoid diabetes or worsening of the fatty liver. An important aspect of my treatment for all of my conditions is lifestyle changes (i.e. healthy diet, exercise, stress control and healthy supplements approved by my doctor).

My Experience with Hypothyroid Related Emotions

As I began developing hypothyroidism from autoimmune thyroid disease (Hashimoto's), I began having severe anxiety and panic attacks. Many patients experience these, just as the thyroid gland begins to fail and become hypothyroid (depression is also common). With Grave's Disease patients (Autoimmune-Hyperthyroidism), they-too will have the anxiety symptoms but many times these are continuous, until they can begin treatment to slow-down the overproduction of hormone by their thyroid glands.

My anxiety was intermittent and would alternate with spells of depression. Researchers describe anxiety symptoms from autoimmune hypothyroidism, as sometimes being caused by the gland's attempt to "sputter back to life" as it begins to fail in attempt to fight off the autoimmune attack. The actual medical term for this is "Hashitoxicosis" (short-term phases of hyperthyroidism) and patients will have it to varying degrees but it usually manifests in a milder form that can still cause significant anxiety symptoms. Milder flares might be better-termed as "thyroiditis flares" because true Hashitoxicosis would cause significant, long-term hyperthyroidism.

Following is a quote from Richard C. W. Hall, M.D., who points out the fact that anxiety is a common symptom found in newly diagnosed hypothyroid patients:

"The development of severe anxiety disorders in hypothyroid states are as much or more related to the rapidity of change of thyroid hormone levels as they are to the absolute levels encountered.

Whether the cause of hypothyroidism is auto-immune or follows thyroidectomy, oblation of the gland by radioactive iodine, the ingestion of medicines such as lithium carbonate, or is associated with thyroid cancer, the neuropsychiatric symptoms are similar."

(From the Research Article Titled: "ANXIETY AND ENDOCRINE DISEASE" - Online Link Location: http://www.drrichardhall.com/anxiety.htm)

Symptoms of Anxiety

What are the symptoms of anxiety that can be experienced by thyroid patients? Following are some of the more common symptoms of anxiety in-general.

- sudden intense feelings of fear

- rapid heart rate

- elevated blood pressure

- rapid breathing (hyperventilation)

- sweating

- trembling

- muscle tension with pain (including chest area)

There can also be anxiety that is more of a constant type keyed-up feeling, called "free floating anxiety" that causes a continuous nervous feeling and one of being on-edge that thyroid patients can experience. This also brings on feelings of constant, chronic worry that is referred to as "Generalized Anxiety Disorder". The more intense episodes of anxiety come under the heading of "anxiety attacks" and "panic attacks". These obviously are very unpleasant and there were times I would experience these with my Hashimoto's disease, especially during the night, causing me to awaken in a cold sweat, while I also experienced other hyperthyroid type symptoms, including teporary weight loss from short-term Hashitoxicosis.

Symptoms of Depression

There are symptoms of depression that are common to thyroid disease patients as well, especially prior to being treated. The more common symptoms are:

- feeling slowed down

- inability to enjoy things

- sadness

- irritability

- anger

- feelings of hopelessness (sometimes including suicidal thoughts)

- feeling tired and lethargic

The symptoms of depression can co-exist with anxiety or sometimes will alternate so that a thyroid patient experiences anxiety part of the time and depression part of the time.

My emotional symptoms were some of the first to resolve with thyroid hormone replacement therapy. I still have occasional mild to moderate flares of anxiety and depression symptoms due to having the autoimmune thyroid disease but the improvements over my pre-treatment state have been significant.

Thyroid patients suffering emotional symptoms should be encouraged to know that hormone replacement therapy can potentially improve these symptoms significantly. If it does not do-so adequately in some patients, there are additional medication-options out there that are effective in treating emotional symptoms as well (i.e. antidepressant and anti-anxiety drugs). Psychiatric therapies can also be helpful, such as "Cognitive Behavioral Therapy" and can be combined with drug therapies or administered as stand-alone treatments, depending on the needs of individual hypothyroid patients.

If you suspect that you might have hypothyroidism or hyperthyroidism, it is important that you see a qualified medical doctor for further evaluation. As is the case with most health disorders and diseases, treatments can be more effective and can prevent further complications, the sooner a diagnosis is made and treatment is started.

(END)

Printed in Great Britain
by Amazon